LOW IODINE COOKBOOK

MAIN COURSE – 80 + Low-Iodine Breakfast, Main Course, Dessert and Snacks Recipes

TABLE OF CONTENTS

BREAKFAST 7
Fruit Shake 7
APPLE OATS 8
FRUIT SMOOTHIE 9
OATMEAL 10
BAKED EGG WHITES OATMEAL 11
GREEN SMOOTHIE 12
GRANOLA OATS 13
HOMEMADE GRANOLA 14
GRIDDLE CAKE 15
BANANA GRIDDLE CAKE 16
STARBERRY GRIDDLE CAKE 17
LOW IODINE PANCAKES 19
LOW IODINE STRAWBERRY PANCAKES 20
WAFFLES 21
CREPES 22
OMELLETE 23
AVOCADO OMELLETE 24
EGG AND POTATO BREAKFAST 25
EGG WHITE FRITTATA AND ASPARAGUS BREAKFAST 26
FRIED EGGS 27

LUNCH 29
CROCKPOT CHICKEN STOCK 29
POLLO CON ARROZ 30
ROTINI WITH ZUCCHINI 31

RED CURRY WITH VEGETABLES 32

CHICKEN FAJITA STREET TACOS 33

CAVATAPPI WITH RAPINI 35

STRAWBERRY SANDWICH 36

GUACAMOLE SALAD 37

SPAGHETTI FRITTATA 38

HOME FRIES 39

LOW IODINE SPAGHETTI CARBONARA 40

SPAGHETTI TOMATO SAUCE 41

ROSEMARY CHICKEN CUTLETS WITH CILANTRO 43

ROSEMARY ROASTED TURKEY 44

STUFFED JALAPENOS 45

CABBAGE WRAPPED PORK 46

POTATO AND BEAN EMPANADAS 48

LOW IODINE PIZZA 49

VEGGIE STUFFED MEATBALLS 51

RED ONION PICKLES 52

DINNER 53

MEATLESS FRITTATA 53

TOMATO PASTA SAUCE 54

NOODLE SALAD 55

BROCCOLI CRUSTLESS QUICHE 57

CHEESE AND PESTO TART 58

SALMON PIZZA 59

PORK ASIAN SALAD 61

CHILI PRAWN FRY 62

ZUCCHINI LASAGNE 63

TACO SALAD 64

BEEF AND BARLEY SOUP 66

CHICKEN ENCHILADA SOUP 67

ASIAN CABBAGE SALAD 68

LEMON GARLIC SALAD DRESSING 69

CITRUS SALAD 70

CUCUMBER SALAD 71

THAI CUCUMBER SALAD 72

LENTIL SOUP 73

SAMOSA SOUP 74

VEGETABLE GUMBO 76

DESSERTS & SNACKS 78

THE SIXER JUICE 78

MANGO & WATERMELON SMOOTHIE 79

GREEN SUMMER SMOOTHIE 80

FRUITY SMOOTHIE 81

LIME SMOOTHIE 82

CARROT SMOOTHIE 83

FRUIT CREAM 84

CINNAMON BALLS 85

TOMATO DIP 86

GUACAMOLE 87

LID BROWNIES 88

CHOCOLATE CHIP COOKIES 89

VANILLA CAKE 90

CHOCOLATE FROSTING	91
POPCORN	92
NO BAKE COOKIES	93
BLUEBERRY MUFFIN	94
CARROT MUFFINS	95
PEANUT BUTTER COOKIES	97
BLUEBERRY CRUMBLE	98

☞ Copyright 2018 by Noah Jerris - All rights reserved.

This document is geared towards providing exact and reliable information in regards to the topic and issue covered. The publication is sold with the idea that the publisher is not required to render accounting, officially permitted, or otherwise, qualified services. If advice is necessary, legal or professional, a practiced individual in the profession should be ordered.

- From a Declaration of Principles which was accepted and approved equally by a Committee of the American Bar Association and a Committee of Publishers and Associations.

In no way is it legal to reproduce, duplicate, or transmit any part of this document in either electronic means or in printed format. Recording of this publication is strictly prohibited and any storage of this document is not allowed unless with written permission from the publisher. All rights reserved.

The information provided herein is stated to be truthful and consistent, in that any liability, in terms of inattention or otherwise, by any usage or abuse of any policies, processes, or directions contained within is the solitary and utter responsibility of the recipient reader. Under no circumstances will any legal responsibility or blame be held against the publisher for any reparation, damages, or monetary loss due to the information herein, either directly or indirectly.

Respective authors own all copyrights not held by the publisher.

The information herein is offered for informational purposes solely, and is universal as so. The presentation of the information is without contract or any type of guarantee assurance.

The trademarks that are used are without any consent, and the publication of the trademark is without permission or backing by the trademark owner. All trademarks and brands within this book are for clarifying purposes only and are the owned by the owners themselves, not affiliated with this document.

Introduction

Low Iodine recipes for personal enjoyment but also for family enjoyment. You will love them for sure for how easy it is to prepare them.

BREAKFAST

Fruit Shake

Serves: *1*
Prep Time: *5* Minutes
Cook Time: *5* Minutes
Total Time: *10* Minutes

INGREDIENTS

- 1 banana
- 1 cup orange juice
- 1 cup water
- ½ ice cubes

DIRECTIONS

1. **Place all ingredients in a blender and blend until smooth**
2. **Pour in a glass and serve**

APPLE OATS

Serves: *1*

Prep Time: *5* Minutes

Cook Time: *5* Minutes

Total Time: *10* Minutes

INGREDIENTS

- 1 cup boiling water
- ½ cup apple cider
- 1 apple
- ¾ cup steel cut oats
- cinnamon

DIRECTIONS

1. Boil apples and add steel cut oats and simmer
2. Top cinnamon or raisins and serve

FRUIT SMOOTHIE

Serves: *1*

Prep Time: *5* Minutes

Cook Time: *5* Minutes

Total Time: *10* Minutes

INGREDIENTS

- 1 cup orange juice
- 1 tablespoon egg whites
- ½ banana
- 1 handful frozen strawberries

DIRECTIONS

1. Place all ingredients in a blender and blend until smooth
2. Pour in a glass and serve

OATMEAL

Serves: **1**

Prep Time: **5** Minutes

Cook Time: **5** Minutes

Total Time: **10** Minutes

INGREDIENTS

- 1 apple
- ½ cup oatmeal
- ¼ water
- sugar

DIRECTIONS

1. In a bowl mix all ingredients and pour water
2. Microwave for 2-3 minutes
3. Add sugar and serve

BAKED EGG WHITES OATMEAL

Serves: *1*
Prep Time: *10* Minutes
Cook Time: *10* Minutes
Total Time: *20* Minutes

INGREDIENTS

- 3 egg whites
- ½ cup oil
- 1 cup sugar
- 2 cups oatmeal
- 1 cup milk substitute

DIRECTIONS

1. In a bowl mix all ingredients
2. Bake for 20-25 minutes at 375 F
3. Remove from oven and serve

GREEN SMOOTHIE

Serves: **1**

Prep Time: **5** Minutes

Cook Time: **5** Minutes

Total Time: **10** Minutes

INGREDIENTS

- 5 oz. apple juice
- ¼ cup chopped kale
- ½ cup mango
- ½ pineapple

DIRECTIONS

1. In a blender add all ingredients and blend until smooth
2. Pour into a glass and serve

GRANOLA OATS

Serves: 2

Prep Time: 10 Minutes

Cook Time: 60 Minutes

Total Time: 70 Minutes

INGREDIENTS

- 2 cups oats
- ½ cup brown sugar
- ¼ cup whole flaxseeds
- 2 tsp cinnamon
- ½ cup canola oil
- ½ cup honey
- 1 cup raisins

DIRECTIONS

1. In a bowl mix sugar, flax seeds, oats, cinnamon and set aside
2. In another bowl mix honey, oil and pour into oats mixture

3. Bake at 275 F for 60 minutes
4. Remove and serve

HOMEMADE GRANOLA

Serves: 2
Prep Time: 10 Minutes
Cook Time: 60 Minutes
Total Time: 70 Minutes

INGREDIENTS

- 3 cups oats
- ¼ tsp cinnamon
- ½ tsp nutmeg
- ¼ cup honey
- ¾ cooking oil

DIRECTIONS

1. In a bowl mix nutmeg, oats, salt, cinnamon and set aside

2. In another bowl mix honey oil and pour pour over oats mixture
3. Bake for 60 minutes at 275 F
4. Remove and serve

GRIDDLE CAKE

Serves: 2

Prep Time: 10 Minutes

Cook Time: 30 Minutes

Total Time: 40 Minutes

INGREDIENTS

- 2 tablespoons sugar
- 1 tsp vanilla
- 1 cup flour
- 1 tsp baking powder
- 1 tsp salt
- 1 tsp cinnamon
- 1 tsp vegetable oil
- 2 egg whites

DIRECTIONS

1. In a bowl mix 2 egg whites with all the ingredients
2. Stir until the batter is well mixed
3. Spoon batter onto griddle, make about 6-8 griddle cakes
4. Serve with jam or maple syrup

BANANA GRIDDLE CAKE

Serves: 2
Prep Time: **10** Minutes

Cook Time: **30** Minutes

Total Time: **40** Minutes

INGREDIENTS

- 1 banana
- 2 tablespoons sugar
- 1 tsp vanilla
- 1 cup flour
- 1 tsp baking powder

- 1 tsp salt
- 1 tsp cinnamon
- 1 tsp vegetable oil
- 2 egg whites

DIRECTIONS

1. In a bowl mix 2 egg whites with all the ingredients
2. Stir until the batter is well mixed
3. Spoon batter onto griddle, make about 6-8 griddle cakes
4. Serve with jam or maple syrup

STARBERRY GRIDDLE CAKE

Serves: *2*

Prep Time: *10* Minutes

Cook Time: *30* Minutes

Total Time: *40* Minutes

INGREDIENTS

- 1 handful strawberries
- 2 tablespoons sugar
- 1 tsp vanilla
- 1 cup flour
- 1 tsp baking powder
- 1 tsp salt
- 1 tsp cinnamon
- 1 tsp vegetable oil
- 2 egg whites

DIRECTIONS

1. In a bowl mix 2 egg whites with all the ingredients
2. Stir until the batter is well mixed
3. Spoon batter onto griddle, make about 6-8 griddle cakes
4. Serve with jam or maple syrup

LOW IODINE PANCAKES

Serves: *4*
Prep Time: *10* Minutes
Cook Time: *10* Minutes
Total Time: *20* Minutes

INGREDIENTS

- 2 egg whites
- ¾ tsp salt
- 1 tsp cinnamon
- 1 tsp vegetable oil
- ¾ cup water
- ¼ banana
- 2 tablespoons sugar
- 1 tsp vanilla
- 1 cup flour
- 1 tsp baking powder

DIRECTIONS

1. In a bowl mix all ingredients
2. Pour mixture into a pan and fry 1-2 minutes per side

LOW IODINE STRAWBERRY PANCAKES

Serves: **4**

Prep Time: **10** Minutes

Cook Time: **10** Minutes

Total Time: **20** Minutes

INGREDIENTS

- 2 egg whites
- 1 handful strawberries
- ¾ tsp salt
- 1 tsp cinnamon
- 1 tsp vegetable oil
- ¾ cup water
- ¼ banana
- 2 tablespoons sugar
- 1 tsp vanilla
- 1 cup flour
- 1 tsp baking powder

DIRECTIONS

1. **In a bowl mix all ingredients**

2. Pour mixture into a pan and fry 1-2 minutes per side
3. Remove and serve

WAFFLES

Serves: *4*

Prep Time: *10* Minutes

Cook Time: *10* Minutes

Total Time: *20* Minutes

INGREDIENTS

- 1 cup all-purpose flour
- 1 tsp cinnamon
- 1 tablespoon sugar
- 1 tsp baking powder
- ¼ tsp salt
- ¼ cup water
- ½ cup egg whites
- 1 tablespoon coconut oil

DIRECTIONS

1. In a bowl mix sugar, baking powder, cinnamon, flour and salt
2. In another bowl mix coconut oil, egg, water and add to the flour mixture and stir
3. Pour mixture into waffle iron and cook following manufacturer's instructions
4. Remove and serve

CREPES

Serves: **4**

Prep Time: **10** Minutes

Cook Time: **10** Minutes

Total Time: **20** Minutes

INGREDIENTS

- 0,5 cup coconut milk
- 0,5 cup white flour
- 1 egg white
- 1 tablespoon sugar
- vegetable oil

DIRECTIONS

1. In a bowl mix all dry ingredients
2. Add milk and stir
3. Pour mixture into a pan and cook 30-60 seconds per side
4. Remove and serve with jam

OMELLETE

Serves: 2

Prep Time: 10 Minutes

Cook Time: 10 Minutes

Total Time: 20 Minutes

INGREDIENTS

- ½ cup egg whites
- 1 tablespoon green onions
- 1 tablespoon tomato
- 1 tablespoon cilantro

DIRECTIONS

1. Mix all ingredients in a bowl

2. Pour mixture into a pan and fry for 2-3 minutes per side
3. Remove and serve

AVOCADO OMELLETE

Serves: 2
Prep Time: 10 Minutes
Cook Time: 10 Minutes
Total Time: 20 Minutes

INGREDIENTS

- ½ cup egg whites
- 1 avocado
- 1 tablespoon green onions
- 1 tablespoon tomato
- 1 tablespoon cilantro

DIRECTIONS

1. Mix all ingredients in a bowl

2. Pour mixture into a pan and fry for 2-3 minutes per side
3. Remove and serve

EGG AND POTATO BREAKFAST

Serves: 2

Prep Time: 10 Minutes

Cook Time: 10 Minutes

Total Time: 20 Minutes

INGREDIENTS

- 1 tsp canola oil
- green pepper
- 2 egg whites
- 1 baked potato
- onion

DIRECTIONS

1. In a skillet heat canola oil
2. Cut baked potato into small pieces

3. In a bowl mix all ingredients and place in the skillet
4. Cook until done, remove and serve

EGG WHITE FRITTATA AND ASPARAGUS BREAKFAST

Serves: **4**

Prep Time: **10** Minutes

Cook Time: **30** Minutes

Total Time: **40** Minutes

INGREDIENTS

- 1 tsp canola oil
- green pepper
- 2 egg whites
- 1 baked potato
- onion
- 1 package asparagus

DIRECTIONS

1. **In a skillet heat canola oil**

2. Cut baked potato into small pieces
3. In a bowl mix all ingredients and place in the skillet
4. Cook until done, remove and serve

FRIED EGGS

Serves: 4

Prep Time: 10 Minutes

Cook Time: 30 Minutes

Total Time: 40 Minutes

INGREDIENTS

- 3 slices bread
- 2 egg whites
- non-iodized salt

DIRECTIONS

1. Make a hole into your bread slices
2. Beat egg whites with salt and

3. Place slices in a skillet and pour egg white mixture
4. Cook until done, remove and serve

LUNCH

CROCKPOT CHICKEN STOCK

Serves: **4**

Prep Time: **10** Minutes

Cook Time: **10** Minutes

Total Time: **20** Minutes

INGREDIENTS

- Chicken bones
- 1 stalk celery
- 2 cloves garlic
- 2 bay leaves
- 1 tablespoon pepper corns
- ½ onion
- 1 carrot

DIRECTIONS

1. Cook chicken in the crockpot, remove the meat from bones to the crockpot
2. Add onion, carrot, celery, garlic cloves, peppercorns, bay leaves and fill crockpot with water

3. Cook on low for 7-8 hours
4. Season with non-iodized salt
5. Remove and serve

POLLO CON ARROZ

Serves: **4**
Prep Time: **10** Minutes
Cook Time: **40** Minutes
Total Time: **50** Minutes

INGREDIENTS

- 2 lbs. whole chicken
- ½ cup canola oil
- 1 cup white rice
- ½ onion
- 1 clove garlic
- 1 can no salt tomato sauce
- 1 tsp black pepper

DIRECTIONS

1. Rinse the chicken and pat dry with paper towel
2. In a pan heat oil over medium heat, cook the chi until browned on both sides
3. Transfer to a place, add rice, garlic and onion to the pan
4. Stir constantly until the onion is soft, stir in the tomato sauce, 2 cups water and season with pepper
5. Return the chicken to the pan
6. Reduce heat to low and simmer for 30 minutes
7. When ready, remove and serve

ROTINI WITH ZUCCHINI

Serves: *4*

Prep Time: *10* Minutes

Cook Time: *30* Minutes

Total Time: *40* Minutes

INGREDIENTS

- ½ lb. rotini
- ½ tsp dried basil
- 2 tablespoons olive oil

- 3 cloves garlic
- 2 zucchini
- 1 12 oz. no salt diced tomatoes

DIRECTIONS

1. In a skillet heat oil over medium heat, add zucchini, garlic, tomatoes and sauté for a couple of minutes
2. Add the drained pasta and stir to combine, season with basil, pepper and cook until the pasta is done
3. Remove and serve

RED CURRY WITH VEGETABLES

Serves: *4*
Prep Time: *10*   Minutes

Cook Time: *20*   Minutes

Total Time: *30*   Minutes

INGREDIENTS

- 2 tablespoons red curry paste
- 1 12 oz. can coconut oil

- 1 onion
- 1 bell pepper
- 1 can bamboo shoots
- 2 cups green beans
- 3 oz. mushrooms
- 1 tablespoon sugar
- fresh Thai basil

DIRECTIONS

1. In a skillet, whisk the curry into the coconut milk
2. Add sugar, veggies and cool on low heat
3. Season the curry and sprinkle with Thai basil and cilantro leaves
4. Remove and serve

CHICKEN FAJITA STREET TACOS

Serves: 4
Prep Time: 10 Minutes
Cook Time: 20 Minutes
Total Time: 30 Minutes

INGREDIENTS

- ¾ lb. chicken breast
- 1 onion
- salsa
- Spice mix
- 1 green bell pepper
- 1 tablespoon canola oil
- corn tortillas
- cilantro

DIRECTIONS

1. In a skillet heat oil over medium heat, add onions, chicken and bell pepper
2. Season with spice mix and cook until chicken is tender
3. In an iron skillet over medium heat add heat tortillas
4. Take a tortilla and add chicken and vegetable mixture inside
5. Top with cilantro and onion
6. Serve with salsa

CAVATAPPI WITH RAPINI

Serves: **4**

Prep Time: **10** Minutes

Cook Time: **30** Minutes

Total Time: **40** Minutes

INGREDIENTS

- 1 bunch of rapini
- ½ lb. cavatappi
- 2 tablespoons olive oil
- 2 cloves garlic
- ½ tsp red pepper flakes
- ½ cup wine
- 1 tomato chopped

DIRECTIONS

1. In a saucepan boil rapini and set aside
2. In a pot cook pasta
3. In a skillet heat olive oil over medium heat, add garlic, red pepper flakes, rapini, wine and tomato
4. Bring to boil, stir to combine and cook for another 2-3 minutes

5. Optional season with non-iodized salt, pepper and serve

STRAWBERRY SANDWICH

Serves: *1*

Prep Time: *5* Minutes

Cook Time: *5* Minutes

Total Time: *10* Minutes

INGREDIENTS

- low sodium bread
- apple carrot sticks
- Low sugar strawberry jelly

DIRECTIONS

1. Over place bread put strawberry jelly, and carrot sticks
2. Serve when ready

GUACAMOLE SALAD

Serves: 2
Prep Time: 10 Minutes
Cook Time: 10 Minutes
Total Time: 20 Minutes

INGREDIENTS

- Arugula
- lime juice
- 1 tomatoes
- fresh cilantro
- 1 avocado
- 2 tablespoons onion
- 1 garlic clove
- 1 tsp cumin

DIRECTIONS

1. In a bowl mix all salad ingredients
2. Serve when ready

SPAGHETTI FRITTATA

Serves: **4**

Prep Time: **10** Minutes

Cook Time: **20** Minutes

Total Time: **30** Minutes

INGREDIENTS

- 8 eggs
- 1 tablespoon olive oil
- 1 onion
- 1 bunch fresh spinach
- 2 oz. tomatoes
- 1 clove garlic
- ½ tsp salt
- ½ tsp black pepper
- ¼ lb. spaghetti
- 1 oz. parmesan cheese

DIRECTIONS

1. In a bowl separate 4 of the egg whites and add the remaining 4 whole eggs to the bowl and whisk to combine, set aside

2. Heat oil in a frying pan over medium heat, add onion and cook for 3-4 minutes
3. Add spinach, garlic, tomatoes, pepper and cook for 2-3 minutes
4. Add pasta, pour the eggs and vegetables, lower the heat and cook for another 8-10 minutes
5. Sprinkle with cheese and remove to a plate
6. Top with parmesan and serve

HOME FRIES

Serves: 2

Prep Time: *10* Minutes

Cook Time: *30* Minutes

Total Time: *40* Minutes

INGREDIENTS

- 2 potatoes
- pepper
- non-iodized salt
- olive oil

ECTIONS

    potatoes and place on a cookie sheet
2. Drizzle with olive oil and sprinkle with non-iodized salt and pepper
3. Cook for 20-25 minutes at 375 F
4. Remove and serve

LOW IODINE SPAGHETTI CARBONARA

Serves: 2
Prep Time: 10 Minutes

Cook Time: 20 Minutes

Total Time: 30 Minutes

INGREDIENTS

- 1 box spaghetti
- cilantro
- egg whites
- portobello mushrooms
- ½ onion

- 2 garlic cloves
- olive oil pepper
- oregano
- parsley

DIRECTIONS

1. Boil pasta al dente for 8-10 minutes
2. In a pan pour olive oil and add onion, garlic, oregano, parsley, pepper, cilantro and mushrooms and let them simmer
3. Add wine and cook until is fully evaporated
4. Rinse spaghetti out of boiling water
5. Place spaghetti into a pan and the rest of ingredients over medium heat
6. Pour egg whites and mix with spaghetti
7. Remove and serve

SPAGHETTI TOMATO SAUCE

Serves: 2
Prep Time: *10* Minutes
Cook Time: *10* Minutes

Total Time: *20* Minutes

INGREDIENTS

- 1 20 oz. can tomatoes
- oregano
- 1 5 oz. can tomato paste
- 1 onion
- red pepper
- pepper
- cilantro
- basil
- parsley
- 4 garlic cloves
- olive oil

DIRECTIONS

1. In a casserole heat olive oil, add garlic, onion and cook on medium heat
2. When tender, add the rest of ingredients and cook for 25-30 minutes
3. Add sauce to pasta and serve

ROSEMARY CHICKEN CUTLETS WITH CILANTRO

Serves: *4*

Prep Time: *10* Minutes

Cook Time: *20* Minutes

Total Time: *30* Minutes

INGREDIENTS

- Chicken breast cutlets
- olive oil
- vinegar
- oregano
- ½ onion
- cilantro
- pepper
- Whole wheat organic flour
- Fresh rosemary
- 1 cup basmati rice

DIRECTIONS

1. In a rice cook cook Basmati rice, ad water and cover
2. Season chicken cutlets with pepper and non-iodized salt

3. On a place pour organic flour, oregano and pepper, mix with chicken cutlets until fully covered
4. Place chicken cutlets in a pan and cook over medium heat, sprinkle rosemary
5. When ready remove and serve with Basmati rice

ROSEMARY ROASTED TURKEY

Serves: **4**

Prep Time: **20** Minutes

Cook Time: **240** Minutes

Total Time: **260** Minutes

INGREDIENTS

- ¾ cup olive oil
- 1 tablespoon Italian seasoning
- 1 tsp black pepper
- 2 tablespoons garlic
- 2 tablespoons chopped rosemary
- 1 tablespoon basil
- 1 tsp non-iodized salt

- 1 whole turkey

DIRECTIONS

1. Preheat oven to 300 F
2. In a bowl mix all ingredients except turkey
3. Spread the rosemary mixture over the turkey
4. Rub every portion of the turkey with the mixture
5. Place turkey in the oven and cook for 3 hours on low heat at 180 F
6. Remove and serve

STUFFED JALAPENOS

Serves: 2
Prep Time: **20** Minutes
Cook Time: **20** Minutes
Total Time: **40** Minutes

INGREDIENTS

- 1 lb. pork sausage

- 1 cup Parmesan cheese
- 1 lb. jalapeno peppers
- 1 8 oz. ranch dressing
- 1 8 oz. cream cheese

DIRECTIONS

1. Preheat oven to 400 F
2. In a skillet place sausage over medium heat and cook until brown
3. In another bowl mix parmesan cheese, cream cheese and spoon 1 tablespoon mixture into each jalapeno half
4. Bake for 20 minutes ur until bubbly
5. Remove and serve

CABBAGE WRAPPED PORK

Serves: *4*
Prep Time: *10* Minutes
Cook Time: *30* Minutes
Total Time: *40* Minutes

INGREDIENTS

- 1 cabbage
- 1 tablespoon ginger
- ½ tsp non-iodized salt
- 1 egg white
- 1 lb. pork
- ½ zucchini
- 1 green onion

DIRECTIONS

1. Place the cabbage heat in pot and fill with water, bring to boil
2. Place leaves in a colander, rinse with water
3. In a bowl mix the remaining ingredient
4. Mold each leaf like a cup and fill with a tablespoon of filling
5. Fill the bottom of a wok with water and place steamer into the wok
6. Bring to boil and place the "cups" there for 25 minutes
7. When ready, remove and serve

POTATO AND BEAN EMPANADAS

Serves: 8

Prep Time: 10 Minutes

Cook Time: 20 Minutes

Total Time: 30 Minutes

INGREDIENTS

- 2 cups flour
- ½ tsp salt-free garlic powder
- ½ tsp dried dill
- ½ cup olive oil
- ½ cup cold water
- 1 tablespoon cider vinegar
- 1 egg
- ½ tsp cumin powder
- ½ tsp clove
- ½ tsp red chili pepper flakes
- 1 cup mashed potatoes
- 1 cup black beans
- ½ cup fresh cilantro

DIRECTIONS

1. Into a bowl place flour, vinegar, garlic powder, oil, water and 1 beaten egg, mix until well combine
2. In another bowl mix clove, cumin, chili pepper flakes, potato beans, cilantro and set aside
3. Meanwhile preheat oven to 400 F
4. Divide dough into 8-12 portions and roll each portion into a ball
5. Place 2-3 tablespoons of potato filling into the dough and fold the dough over the filling
6. Place the empanada on a baking sheet and bake for 15-20 minutes or until golden brown
7. Remove and serve

LOW IODINE PIZZA

Serves: 2

Prep Time: 10 Minutes

Cook Time: 20 Minutes

Total Time: 30 Minutes

INGREDIENTS

- Chickpea pizza crust
- Pesto
- Thinly sliced zucchini
- Low-sodium greet yogurt
- Low-sodium Swiss cheese
- Mozzarella
- Shredded chicken
- 4-5 slices of lemon
- 4-5 slices jalapenos
- hers

DIRECTIONS

1. Take the chickpea pizza crust
2. Place all the ingredients over the pizza crust
3. Place in the oven for 12-15 minutes at 350 F or until golden brown
4. Remove and serve

VEGGIE STUFFED MEATBALLS

Serves: *12*
Prep Time: *10* Minutes
Cook Time: *30* Minutes
Total Time: *40* Minutes

INGREDIENTS

- 1 zucchini
- 1 lb. pork
- 3 cloves garlic
- 2 green onions

DIRECTIONS

1. Preheat oven to 375 F
2. In a blender add zucchini, garlic, pork and onions, blend until smooth
3. Remove mixture and place meat balls
4. Place on a parchment-covered pan and bake for 25-30 minutes
5. Remove and serve

RED ONION PICKLES

Serves: **4**

Prep Time: **10** Minutes

Cook Time: **30** Minutes

Total Time: **40** Minutes

INGREDIENTS

- 1 onion
- 1 clove garlic
- ¾ cup wine vinegar
- ½ tsp sugar
- ½ tsp salt-free garlic powder
- ½ tsp turmeric

DIRECTIONS

1. In a pot bring 2 cups of water to boil
2. Add garlic powder, turmeric, sugar and vinegar
3. Cook until sugar dissolved
4. In a jar place onions and pour pickling liquid over, close the jar
5. Drain onion before using

DINNER

MEATLESS FRITTATA

Serves: **4**

Prep Time: **10** Minutes

Cook Time: **50** Minutes

Total Time: **60** Minutes

INGREDIENTS

- 8 eggs
- 1 cup milk
- 5 onions
- ½ bunch parsley
- ½ corn kernels
- ¼ lb. olives
- 1 jar roasted peppers
- ½ lb. cheese
- 1 lb. Turkish bread

DIRECTIONS

1. **Preheat oven to 300 F**
2. **In a bowl mix milk and eggs together**

3. Stir in corn, olives, cheese, pepper, parsley and onions
4. Add the bread and stir
5. Cook for 40-45 minutes
6. Remove, allow to cool and serve

TOMATO PASTA SAUCE

Serves: 2
Prep Time: 5 Minutes
Cook Time: 5 Minutes
Total Time: 10 Minutes

INGREDIENTS

- 1 bunch herbs
- 1 lb. tomatoes
- 1 lb. tin tomatoes
- 1 pinch chili flakes
- 1/3 lb. water
- 1/3 lb. tomato paste
- 1 tsp sugar
- 3 cloves garlic

- 1 onion
- 1 carrot
- 1 oz. olive oil

DIRECTIONS

1. In a blender place all the ingredients and blend until smooth
2. Pour smoothie into a glass and serve

NOODLE SALAD

Serves: *4*

Prep Time: *10* Minutes

Cook Time: *20* Minutes

Total Time: *30* Minutes

INGREDIENTS

- 2 leftover cooked chicken legs
- 1 red Chilli
- 1 inch. piece ginger

- 1 tablespoon soy sauce
- 1 tablespoon rice vinegar
- 1 spring onion
- 1 tablespoon coriander
- ½ lb. noodles
- ½ tsp wasabi
- 1 tsp sesame oil

DIRECTIONS

1. In a pan boil water and add noodles
2. In a jar mix vinegar, wasabi, ginger, soy sauce and sesame oil
3. Toss the noodles wit the dressing and let it stand for 15-20 minutes
4. Arrange noodles in a bowl, top with chicken, onions and coriander and serve

BROCCOLI CRUSTLESS QUICHE

Serves: **6**

Prep Time: **10** Minutes

Cook Time: **50** Minutes

Total Time: **60** Minutes

INGREDIENTS

- 1 onion
- 3 oz. raising flour
- 1 lb. broccoli florets
- 1 red capsicum
- 1/3 lb. cheddar cheese
- 1.5 oz. parmesan cheese
- 3 eggs
- 1 lb. milk

DIRECTIONS

1. **Preheat oven to 300 f**
2. **In a dish add veggies, onions and grated cheese**
3. **In a bowl mix flour, eggs and whisk to combine, add milk and whisk to combine**

4. Pour mixture into dish and bake for 40 minutes or until golden brown
5. Remove, let it cool and serve

CHEESE AND PESTO TART

Serves: 2
Prep Time: 10 Minutes
Cook Time: 30 Minutes
Total Time: 40 Minutes

INGREDIENTS

- 1 sheet puff pastry
- 1 handful cherry tomatoes
- 1 handful Kalamata olive
- 2 tablespoon kale and basil pesto
- 2,5 oz. cheddar cheese
- 1 tablespoon pine nuts

DIRECTIONS

1. Preheat oven at 300 F and line a baking sheet

2. Place pastry sheet on baking tray, fork the pastry all over the center of the pastry
3. Spread the pesto over the center of the tart, top with tomatoes, olives and top with grated cheese, top with pine nuts
4. Bake for 20 minutes, remove and serve

SALMON PIZZA

Serves: 2

Prep Time: 10 Minutes

Cook Time: 15 Minutes

Total Time: 25 Minutes

INGREDIENTS

- ½ lb. Greek yoghurt
- ½ lb. self raising flour

PIZZA BASE

- ½ cup pasta sauce
- 2 oz. baby spinach
- 1 cup grated mozzarella
- 1/3 lb. smoked salmon

- ½ cup feta

DIRECTIONS

1. Preheat the oven to 300 F
2. In a bowl mix Greek Yogurt and mix flour, transfer to a work surface
3. Grease 2 pizza trays and divide dough in half and spread each one
4. Bake for 4-5 minutes and remove from the oven
5. Cover with tomato sauce, sprinkle spinach leaves, salmon, mozzarella and feta
6. Return to the oven and bake for another 10-12 minutes
7. Remove and serve

PORK ASIAN SALAD

Serves: 2

Prep Time: 10 Minutes

Cook Time: 10 Minutes

Total Time: 20 Minutes

INGREDIENTS

- 1 lb. shredded pork
- ½ red cabbage
- 3 carrots
- 4 onions
- 1 red chili
- ½ bunch coriander

DRESSING

- 3 tablespoons hoisin sauce
- 1 tablespoon sesame oil

DIRECTIONS

1. In a bowl mix all salad ingredients
2. In a jar mix dressing ingredients
3. Pour dressing over salad and serve

CHILI PRAWN FRY

Serves: **4**

Prep Time: **10** Minutes

Cook Time: **20** Minutes

Total Time: **30** Minutes

INGREDIENTS

- 2 carrots
- ¼ lb. snow peas
- 1 tsp olive oil
- 1 garlic clove
- 1 green chili
- 1 tablespoon soy sauce
- 1 tablespoon wine
- 1 tsp sesame oil
- ½ lb. prawns

DIRECTIONS

1. In a wok add oil, garlic, chili, veggies and cook over medium heat for 2-3 minutes
2. In a pan boil noodles

3. Add sesame oil, soy sauce into the wok and cook for 2-3 minutes
4. Add the prawns and fry for 2-3 minutes
5. Serve with noodles

ZUCCHINI LASAGNE

Serves: **4**

Prep Time: **10** Minutes

Cook Time: **30** Minutes

Total Time: **40** Minutes

INGREDIENTS

- 1 tablespoon olive oil
- 1 onion
- 3 garlic cloves
- 1,5 lb. zucchini
- ½ lb. quark
- 2 oz. cheddar cheese
- 1 oz. pizza cheese
- 3 lasagna sheets
- 1 lb. tomato pasta sauce

ECTIONS

1. at oven to 350 F
2. In a frying pan fry onion for 2-3 minutes, add garlic, zucchini, garlic and cook for another 2-3 minutes
3. Stir in 2/3 quark, cheddar cheese and season
4. Heat the tomato sauce and layer up a baking dish, add zucchini mixture, lasagna sheets, tomato sauce and remaining quark
5. Sprinkle the cheddar cheese and pizza cheese
6. Bake for 15-20 minutes or until golden brown
7. Remove and serve

TACO SALAD

Serves: **4**
Prep Time: **10** Minutes
Cook Time: **30** Minutes
Total Time: **40** Minutes

INGREDIENTS

- 1,5 lb. cooked chicken breast

- ½ lb. cherry tomatoes
- 3 onions
- 1 lb. can red kidney
- 1 lb. can corn kernels
- ¼ lb. salsa
- ¼ lb. corn
- ½ avocado
- lime wedges
- ¼ lb. salad leaves
- ½ iceberg lettuce
- 1 red capsicum

DIRECTIONS

1. In a bowl mix all salad ingredients
2. Sprinkle onion over the greens
3. Mix the beans and corn together
4. Top with shredded chicken

BEEF AND BARLEY SOUP

Serves: **6**

Prep Time: **10** Minutes

Cook Time: **250** Minutes

Total Time: **260** Minutes

INGREDIENTS

- 1 lb. stew meat
- 1 onion
- 1 carrot
- 2 russet potatoes
- 3 oz. white mushrooms
- ½ cup barley
- 30 oz. unsalted beef stock
- 1 cup water

DIRECTIONS

1. Place all ingredients in a crockpot
2. Cook on high for 4-5 hours
3. Remove and serve

CHICKEN ENCHILADA SOUP

Serves: **6**

Prep Time: **10** Minutes

Cook Time: **250** Minutes

Total Time: **260** Minutes

INGREDIENTS

- 2 chicken breasts
- 1 jalapeno
- 1 zucchini
- 1 cup corn
- 1 onion
- 12 oz. can no salted tomatoes
- 2 tablespoons chili powder
- 1 tsp cumin
- ½ tsp black pepper
- 6 cups unsalted chicken broth
- ½ cup cilantro
- 2 cloves garlic
- 2 poblano peppers

DIRECTIONS

1. Place all ingredients in a crockpot
2. Cook on high for 4-5 hours
3. Remove and serve

ASIAN CABBAGE SALAD

Serves: **4**

Prep Time: **10** Minutes

Cook Time: **10** Minutes

Total Time: **20** Minutes

INGREDIENTS

- ½ head green cabbage
- 1 cucumber
- 2 cloves garlic
- ½ cup rice vinegar
- 2 tablespoons sugar
- 1 carrot
- 1 fresh Chile
- 2 tablespoons cilantro

DIRECTIONS

1. In a bowl mix all salad ingredients
2. In another bowl mix vinegar, sugar, garlic and pour mixture over salad and serve

LEMON GARLIC SALAD DRESSING

Serves: 2
Prep Time: 5 Minutes
Cook Time: 5 Minutes
Total Time: 10 Minutes

INGREDIENTS

- ½ lemon juice
- ½ cup olive oil
- 1 clove garlic

DIRECTIONS

1. In a jar mix all ingredients
2. Pour dressing over salad and serve

CITRUS SALAD

Serves: **2**

Prep Time: **10** Minutes

Cook Time: **10** Minutes

Total Time: **20** Minutes

INGREDIENTS

- 1 avocado
- 1 tablespoon olive oil
- pepper
- sugar
- 1 grapefruit
- 1 orange
- 1 cup arugula

DIRECTIONS

1. In a bowl mix all salad ingredients
2. Squeeze the juice from the grapefruit over salad and serve

CUCUMBER SALAD

Serves: **2**

Prep Time: **10** Minutes

Cook Time: **10** Minutes

Total Time: **20** Minutes

INGREDIENTS

- 1 cucumber
- ½ onion
- 1 jalapeno
- ½ cup vinegar
- ½ cup water
- 1 tablespoon sugar
- herbs

DIRECTIONS

1. In a bowl mix all salad ingredients
2. In another bowl mix vinegar, sugar and water and pour dressing over salad
3. Season with herbs and serve

THAI CUCUMBER SALAD

Serves: 2
Prep Time: 10 Minutes
Cook Time: 10 Minutes
Total Time: 20 Minutes

INGREDIENTS

- 2 cucumbers
- 1 fresh thai basil leaves
- ½ cup rice vinegar
- ½ cup sugar
- 2 tablespoons water
- ½ onion
- 2 jalapenos
- herbs
- 1 fresh cilantro
- 1 fresh mint leaves

DIRECTIONS

1. In a bowl mix all salad ingredients
2. In another bowl mix sugar, water and rice vinegar

3. Pour dressing over cucumber salad
4. Mix well and serve

LENTIL SOUP

Serves: **4**

Prep Time: **10** Minutes

Cook Time: **40** Minutes

Total Time: **50** Minutes

INGREDIENTS

- 1 tablespoon canola oil
- 1 carrot
- 2 cloves garlic
- 1 tsp cumin
- 1 jalapeno
- 12 oz. can no slat tomatoes
- ½ cup lentils
- 1 onion
- ½ tsp coriander
- 6 cups vegetable broth

- 1 zucchini
- 2 stalks celery

DIRECTIONS

1. In a soup pot heat oil over medium heat
2. Add celery, carrots, onion and cook until tender
3. Add garlic, tomatoes, lentils, jalapeno, coriander, cumin and vegetable broth
4. Bring to simmer and cook for 20-25 minutes
5. Add zucchini and cilantro and cook for another 10-15 minutes
6. Season with pepper and serve

SAMOSA SOUP

Serves: *4*

Prep Time: *10* Minutes

Cook Time: *20* Minutes

Total Time: *30* Minutes

INGREDIENTS

- 2 tsp canola oil
- 1 onion
- 2 cloves garlic
- 1-inch piece ginger
- 1 jalapeno
- 1 tsp curry powder
- dash pepper
- 2 medium potatoes
- ½ cup green split peas
- 6 cups vegetable broth
- ½ cup green peas
- ½ fresh cilantro

DIRECTIONS

1. Heat canola oil in a pot over medium heat
2. Add onions, jalapeno, garlic, ginger and sauté
3. Add pepper, vegetable broth, green split peas, curry powder and cook for 10-12 minutes
4. Add potatoes, green peas, and season, cook for another 5-10 minutes
5. Take off heat add cilantro and serve

VEGETABLE GUMBO

Serves: **4**

Prep Time: **10** Minutes

Cook Time: **60** Minutes

Total Time: **70** Minutes

INGREDIENTS

- ½ cup canola oil
- 1 12 oz. can salt free tomatoes
- 1 32 oz. unsalted chicken broth
- 1 tablespoon parsley
- 1 lb. sliced okra
- ½ tsp dried thyme
- ½ tsp oregano
- ½ cup flour
- ½ tsp black pepper
- ¼ tsp cayenne pepper
- 1 zucchini
- 1 onion
- 1 green bell pepper
- 2 stalks celery

DIRECTIONS

1. In a Dutch oven heat oil and flour over medium heat
2. Add bell pepper, celery, onion, tomatoes, chicken broth, thyme, parsley, pepper, oregano and cook for 10 minutes or until soft
3. Add the okra and simmer for 30 minutes
4. Add zucchini and simmer for another 20 minutes
5. Remove to a place and serve with rice

DESSERTS & SNACKS

THE SIXER JUICE

Serves: 2
Prep Time: 5 Minutes
Cook Time: 5 Minutes
Total Time: 10 Minutes

INGREDIENTS

- 1 mango
- 1 banana
- 1 green apple
- ½ cucumber
- 1 handful of baby spinach leaves
- 1 kiwi
- 1 try ice cubes
- 2 cups water

DIRECTIONS

1. In a blender place all the ingredients and blend until smooth
2. Pour smoothie into a glass and serve

MANGO & WATERMELON SMOOTHIE

Serves: 2

Prep Time: 5 Minutes

Cook Time: 5 Minutes

Total Time: 10 Minutes

INGREDIENTS

- 2 mangoes
- ½ lb. watermelon
- 1-2 tablespoon mint leaves
- 1 tray ice cube

DIRECTIONS

1. In a blender place all the ingredients and blend until smooth
2. Pour smoothie into a glass and serve

GREEN SUMMER SMOOTHIE

Serves: 2
Prep Time: 5 Minutes
Cook Time: 5 Minutes
Total Time: 10 Minutes

INGREDIENTS

- 1 banana
- 1 orange
- 1 apple
- ½ cucumber
- 1 handful of baby spinach
- 1 handful of strawberries
- 1 tray ice cubes
- ½ lb. water

DIRECTIONS

1. In a blender place all the ingredients and blend until smooth
2. Pour smoothie into a glass and serve

FRUITY SMOOTHIE

Serves: **2**

Prep Time: **5** Minutes

Cook Time: **5** Minutes

Total Time: **10** Minutes

INGREDIENTS

- 1 banana
- 1 orange
- 1 apple
- ½ cucumber
- 1 handful of baby spinach
- 1 tray ice cubes
- ½ lb. cold water

DIRECTIONS

1. **In a blender place all the ingredients and blend until smooth**
2. **Pour smoothie into a glass and serve**

LIME SMOOTHIE

Serves: 2
Prep Time: 5 Minutes
Cook Time: 5 Minutes
Total Time: 10 Minutes

INGREDIENTS

- 1 stick celery
- 1 orange
- 1 handful of baby spinach
- juice of ½ lime
- 1-2 tablespoon mint leaves
- 1 tray ice cube

DIRECTIONS

1. In a blender place all the ingredients and blend until smooth
2. Pour smoothie into a glass and serve

CARROT SMOOTHIE

Serves: **2**

Prep Time: **5** Minutes

Cook Time: **5** Minutes

Total Time: **10** Minutes

INGREDIENTS

- 1 carrot
- 2 oranges
- 1-2 tablespoon mint leaves
- 1 tray ice cube

DIRECTIONS

1. In a blender place all the ingredients and blend until smooth
2. Pour smoothie into a glass and serve

FRUIT CREAM

Serves: *2*

Prep Time: *10* Minutes

Cook Time: *10* Minutes

Total Time: *20* Minutes

INGREDIENTS

- 2 oz. sugar
- 2/3 lb. frozen strawberries or any other
- 1 egg white

DIRECTIONS

1. In a blender place all the ingredients and blend until smooth
2. Pour smoothie into a glass and serve

CINNAMON BALLS

Serves: **4**

Prep Time: **10** Minutes

Cook Time: **30** Minutes

Total Time: **40** Minutes

INGREDIENTS

- ½ cup sugar
- 1 egg white
- icing sugar
- ½ lb. almonds
- 1 tsp cinnamon

DIRECTIONS

1. Preheat oven to 300 F
2. In a bowl mix all dry ingredients
3. In another bowl beat the egg and fold in the dry ingredients
4. Bake for 15-20 minutes
5. Remove and allow to cool

TOMATO DIP

Serves: 2
Prep Time: 5 Minutes
Cook Time: 5 Minutes
Total Time: 10 Minutes

INGREDIENTS

- 1 lb. chopped tomatoes
- 1 clove garlic
- 1 onion
- 1tsp Cajun seasoning

DIRECTIONS

1. In a blender place all the ingredients and blend until smooth
2. Pour smoothie into a glass and serve

GUACAMOLE

Serves: **2**

Prep Time: **5** Minutes

Cook Time: **5** Minutes

Total Time: **10** Minutes

INGREDIENTS

- 2 avocado pears
- 1 chili
- 1 clove garlic
- ½ red onion
- ½ lemon

DIRECTIONS

1. In a blender place all the ingredients and blend until smooth
2. Pour smoothie into a glass and serve

LID BROWNIES

Serves: **3**

Prep Time: **10** Minutes

Cook Time: **30** Minutes

Total Time: **40** Minutes

INGREDIENTS

- 1 cup sugar
- ½ tsp baking powder
- ½ tsp salt
- ½ cup chopped nuts
- 3 egg whites
- ½ cup salt-free margarine
- 2 oz. Nestle choco-bake
- 2 tablespoons vegetable oil
- 1 tsp vanilla extract
- 1/3 cup all purpose flour

DIRECTIONS

1. In a bowl mix Nestle choco-bake, egg whites, sugar, margarine and vanilla
2. Add salt, baking powder, flour, nuts and mix well

3. Spread mixture into a baking pan and bake at 325 F for 30 minutes
4. Add chocolate chips and serve

CHOCOLATE CHIP COOKIES

Serves: **4**

Prep Time: **10** Minutes

Cook Time: **20** Minutes

Total Time: **30** Minutes

INGREDIENTS

- 2 sticks softened salt-free margarine
- 1 cup sugar
- 1 tsp vanilla extract
- 3 egg whites
- 2 cups flour
- 1 tsp baking powder
- 1 tsp baking soda
- 1 tsp salt
- 10 oz. salt-free chocolate chips

DIRECTIONS

1. Cream together sugar, egg whites, vanilla and margarine
2. Sift in dry ingredients and mix until completely incorporated
3. Add chocolate chips and bake at 350 F for 10-12 minutes or until golden brown
4. Remove and serve

VANILLA CAKE

Serves: **4**

Prep Time: **10** Minutes

Cook Time: **40** Minutes

Total Time: **50** Minutes

INGREDIENTS

- 2 cups flour
- 1 tsp baking powder
- 1 cup sugar
- 1 cup water

- 1 tsp vanilla
- 3 egg whites
- ½ canola oil

DIRECTIONS

1. In a bowl mix sugar, oil, water, vanilla and egg whites
2. Sift together baking powder and flour, add dry ingredients and stir until fully incorporated
3. Pour into a pan and bake at 325 F for 40 minutes
4. Remove and serve

CHOCOLATE FROSTING

Serves: *4*

Prep Time: *10* Minutes

Cook Time: *10* Minutes

Total Time: *20* Minutes

INGREDIENTS

- 2 cups sugar

- ½ cup boiling water
- 1/3 cup salt-free margarine
- 2 oz. Nestle Choco-bake
- 2 tsp chocolate liquor

DIRECTIONS

1. In a bowl mix sugar with margarine and Choco-bake, microwave until fully melted
2. Add boiling water, vanilla and liquor and let it stand before frosting
3. Frost and serve when ready

POPCORN

Serves: 2
Prep Time: 10 Minutes
Cook Time: 10 Minutes
Total Time: 20 Minutes

INGREDIENTS

- ½ cup kernels
- 3 tablespoons olive oil
- non-iodine salt

DIRECTIONS

1. In a pot over medium heat add olive oil and ½ cup kernels
2. Shake and add the rest of the kernels
3. Add salt, remove and serve

NO BAKE COOKIES

Serves: *4*

Prep Time: *10* Minutes

Cook Time: *10* Minutes

Total Time: *20* Minutes

INGREDIENTS

- ½ cup coconut oil
- ½ cup sugar

- 1 tablespoon vanilla
- 2/4 cup oats
- ½ cup peanut butter
- ½ cup cocoa

DIRECTIONS

1. In a saucepan melt peanut butter and oil
2. When fully melted add sugar and vanilla and stir
3. Add oats and continue stirring
4. Pour onto wax paper and serve

BLUEBERRY MUFFIN

Serves: *4*
Prep Time: *10* Minutes
Cook Time: *30* Minutes
Total Time: *40* Minutes

INGREDIENTS

- 2 egg whites

- ½ cup sugar
- 2 tsp baking powder
- 1 cup blueberries
- 1 cup water
- ½ cup vegetable oil
- 2 cups flour

DIRECTIONS

1. Preheat oven to 375
2. In a bowl mix egg whites, oil and water
3. Add baking powder, sugar and flour and blueberries
4. Pour batter into a muffin pan
5. Bake for 15-20 minutes or until ready at 375 F
6. Remove and serve

CARROT MUFFINS

Serves: **10**

Prep Time: **10** Minutes

Cook Time: **30** Minutes

Total Time: **40** Minutes

INGREDIENTS

- 2 cups flour
- 1 cup carrots
- 1 cup
- 3 egg whites
- ½ cup oil
- 2/4 cup brown sugar
- 1 tsp baking soda
- ½ tsp cinnamon
- 1 cup crushed pineapple

DIRECTIONS

1. In a bowl mix dry ingredients, add beaten egg whites, mix with pineapple, carrots and oil
2. Pour butter into a muffin tin and bake at 375 for 15-20 minutes
3. Remove and serve

PEANUT BUTTER COOKIES

Serves: **4**

Prep Time: **10** Minutes

Cook Time: **30** Minutes

Total Time: **40** Minutes

INGREDIENTS

- 1 cup peanut butter
- 2/3 cup sugar
- 1 tsp baking soda
- 1 tsp flour
- 1 egg white
- 1 tsp vanilla

DIRECTIONS

1. Preheat oven to 350 F
2. In a bowl mix baking soda, flour, peanut butter, sugar, vanilla and egg whites
3. Take dough and roll into balls
4. Bake at 350 for 12-15 minutes, remove and serve

BLUEBERRY CRUMBLE

Serves: **4**

Prep Time: **10** Minutes

Cook Time: **40** Minutes

Total Time: **50** Minutes

INGREDIENTS

- 3 peaches
- ¼ cup blueberries
- ½ cup flour
- ½ cup almonds
- 2 tablespoons sugar
- ½ cup oats
- 1 tablespoon brown sugar
- 2 tablespoons coconut oil

DIRECTIONS

1. Cut the peaches in half, chop the peaches and place in a baking dish
2. Add blueberries, sprinkle with sugar and stir to combine
3. In a bowl mix sugar, oats, flour and almonds

4. Add coconut oil and spread mixture over baking dish
5. Bake at 350 F for 30-35 minutes or until golden brown
6. Remove and serve

Thank you for reading this book!

Printed in Great Britain
by Amazon